WEIGHT LOSS SURGERY NIGHTMARE

SILAS SCOTT

INDEPENDENTLY PUBLISHED

Copyright © 2023 Weight Loss Surgery Nightmare by SILAS SCOTT

All rights reserved.

No part of this book may be reproduced in any form or by any electronic or mechanical means, including information storage and retrieval systems, without written permission from the author, except for the use of brief quotations in a book review.

The ISBN-13 or ASIN number can be located on the back cover of the print books or is on file with the publisher, respectively.

Weight Loss Surgery Nightmare is a memoir. It reflects the personal experiences of the author as he perceived them. The names of people have been changed to protect the identity of anyone referenced or discussed other than public figures.

Dedication

This book is dedicated to my parents, whom took care of me as I struggled through two long and terrifying recoveries after these desperate surgeries.

Your love and support (even when you didn't agree with my choices) literally helped me to survive, and eventually to regain a reasonable quality of life.

So many of the most wonderful events of my life have happened since those horrific times. Thanks for loving me through it all, no matter my shape or size.

INTRODUCTION

I'm not a medical expert, so this book isn't about advice or science. I'm a survivor. This is my story of how two bariatric (or weight-loss) surgeries "ruined" my life; sending me on a rollercoaster ride of crippling disability, physical and mental suffering, fat loss and gain—to my current state—usually fat, mostly happy, and much more experienced and informed about the possible results of surgical interventions for obesity.

PART ONE

I was a skinny kid. A typical child of the 70s. I was never especially interested in food. There were too many interesting things to do.

I liked food—after my parents spent years forcing me to eat. Just a little. As a young child, I just didn't see meals as entertainment or an important source of pleasure. My "always dieting" mom seemed effortlessly thin. My dad was always chubby after my younger brother and I were born. He had a belly. He definitely perceived food as entertainment. The way he gained and carried weight on his body was a premonition of my future. I don't recall him talking about it or even being self-conscious about it. My little brother was a natural athlete and always fit. My paternal grandmother was short and chunky. She liked to nibble while she (continuously) cooked, but I think it was determined mostly by genetic factors. I had a few chubby aunts and uncles (out of many,) but my dozens of cousins, neighborhood friends, and almost all of my classmates were thin or athletic in build—seemingly without much conscious thought or effort. We never talked about it. The exception being the one obese girl in our class whom was ostracized and truly treated as an outcast.

In my early elementary school years, I remember being forced by my teachers to take at least one bite of each type of food on my lunch tray. We had tasty, fattening lunches, so I liked most of what we were served; but it wasn't a lot of food. Meals at home were similar. Nearly everything was homemade and tasted really good. I just wasn't interested. At home, I usually had to eat 2-3 bites of each item on my plate before I could leave the table and "be done."

I didn't care for desserts. My mother held back on the sugar when she made Koolaid. I didn't care for orange juice, and other fruit juices didn't seem to be commonly around back then—at least not in our house. I would drink a little milk (we never had over 2% fat.) Pop aka Pepsi, Coke, RC, etc.; was like a Friday night treat. I loved candy, and had it often, but not in vast amounts.

The snacks I always went for were sliced apples, white bread (carefully folded and eaten in a pattern,) and sliced cheese—also carefully folded for consumption.

On Sundays after church, when every lunch was a family gathering at my grandma's house; my bizarre lack of enthusiasm about food continued. I say it was strange, because my Grams laid out a helluva spread. With many mouths to feed and not much money, the Sunday lunches were always large and eclectic. Nearly always, the main entrée was fried chicken with all the traditional sides, but there would also be an extensive selection of random food to make sure everyone had their fill. While my lean mother was cleaning a few pieces of chicken down to the bone (one of her few weaknesses,) my Grams had her customary cottage cheese with fruit (her method of controlling her diabetes,) my dad and most of the others piled their plates high (often more than once,) but not me.

I would often have a few bites of different dishes, but usually without fail, I had my special—two pieces of white bread, hand torn into tiny morsels to make a pile, which I then covered with homemade white gravy (made with the rendered fat from the chicken.) Sometimes I did mashed potatoes like the others, but mostly—bread and gravy.

I shared that odd food obsession to give you some insight into my early relationship with food. I appreciated the taste, but mostly just ate an amount that met my parents' requirements so that I could return to watching TV while I was sketching, or climbing trees, or reading on the porch swing. Or making a mixed tape with a tape recorder and a radio. Food was MOSTLY just what I had to get through so I could get back to more interesting activities.

Being young, thin, and attractive—in the 70s when guys didn't wear a lot of clothes in the summer (I had several matching midriff shirts and short short sets—they weren't Queer clothes, they were the norm) I got quite a bit of confusing attention. As an introvert who barely had any awareness that sexuality existed, this was perceived by me and others in a number of ways.

First of all, as a pre-adolescent, whom never wore my hair long and wore typical boys' clothes; I still occasionally caught the attention of men in public settings. More than once, strange men told my mom (within my hearing) what a pretty girl I was. I was both excited and horrified to have men look at me that way. In retrospect, it was a bit pervy on their part. In every instance, my mother was immediately angry and indignant. She would correct them regarding my gender and drag me away. I think she was scared for me, insulted by the notion that I didn't present as masculine enough, and deep down—afraid for the future, because she began to sense that I was Gay; though I don't think she probably acknowledged that to herself on any conscious level.

Every day in the summer was spent at the community swimming pool. In fact, that's where all the kids I knew spent their summers. When we were little, my mother often went with us, and she sunbathed as we swam, but by the time we entered middle school, we could go by ourselves. Though not an athlete, I was thin and fit, so summers were spent in nothing but a pair of short, wet swimming trunks.

Though shy and naïve, it was then that I became slightly more sexually aware and conscious of my attraction to men and other boys my age. There were sexy lifeguards, naked guys in the locker room and wet, barely clothed boys climbing all over each other in the water.

Of course, around this time, puberty hit and everything changed. I learned people had sex, what every guy's favorite solitary pastime is, and realized I was Gay.

Being old enough to work to earn my own money soon meant learning that living in a small town surrounded by farmers didn't provide a lot of job opportunities for teens (that weren't hard manual labor.) I didn't enjoy working in the fields doing farmwork, so I turned to my favorite place in town—the swimming pool.

I got a job as a young teen, working in the concession stand and teaching private swimming lessons to little kids. I taught some kids for whom I also babysat.

Babysitting also had an impact on my sexualization—or lack thereof. I say this because the father of the toddlers I babysat for was a sexy young guy that I quickly became infatuated with. On a more dangerous note, I sensed he was sexually interested in me too.

He was young and fit, and his very over-weight wife was kept away much of the time by her busy career as a nurse. I felt guilty about the attraction because she was always very nice to me and treated me with complete trust.

Now, before you start assuming that the dad was a jerk or a child molester, let me assure you that nothing happened. He may have been straight (I don't know. They did divorce years later after having another baby.) I think he was a normal horny man, whom rarely had time with his wife, and may not have been attracted to her after her weight gain (After their divorce, she became a runner and was slim and fit.)

He would come home from work late in the evenings. The kids would already be asleep. I would be sprawled on the living room floor—nearly naked in one of my little 70s era outfits. He would come in and sit down in a chair behind me to "rest for a few minutes" before driving me home.

I could tell without a doubt that if I would initiate sex with him, he would have eagerly done it (although I was about 14 at the time.) I wanted it SO much, but I was shy and completely inexperienced. Looking back, I see I teased him, rolling around on the floor, striking provocative poses. I still fantasize about it to this day—with regret for maybe corrupting him a little, and greater regret that I didn't do it. I think it would have helped be come out of my shell so I could have been brave enough to socialize appropriately with the other closeted boys in town more similar to me in age.

Instead, none of that happened, and I began to subconsciously build a fortress of fat to protect me from having to acknowledge and engage with ANYONE sexually or in a romantic sense. I became very uncomfortable with attention from boys and men because I didn't want to be Gay.

Some guys in high school started to tease and harass me a little in a low-key way. At the time, I was frightened by it (more because of fear of being outed, than thinking any of them would physically harm me.)

It was only years later, when I learned that some of my bullies were Gay or bisexual themselves and actively had secret sex with other guys at the time, that I understood that some of them were actually flirting with me and testing my boundaries and interest.

My internalized homophobia caused me to perceive their flirtation and sexual overtures as harassment and threats. What a waste of time and opportunity. While my straight friends were dating and experimenting with sex, acquiring the confidence necessary for romantic relationships. I could have been doing much the same thing (though secrecy would have been required.) Instead of developing the confidence and self-respect to function as a normal sexual Gay man, all of this pushed me further into the protective bubble of obesity. I started eating for pleasure (because I wasn't going out and socializing with other people,) and with ZERO conscious awareness of it, making myself less physically attractive; so that guys stopped flirting with me and lusting after me. I was safe from having to deal with being a person I didn't want to be.

Looking back, I know now that I wasn't that overweight in high school. I developed a bit of a belly, and my cheeks filled out some; but I no longer had confidence in my appearance.

My hard judgment of my changing body allowed me to stop seeing sex as even an option, and the bigger I became, the more everyone just treated me as asexual. It didn't matter much if I was Gay, because no one was still interested in me anyway.

By the time I graduated from high school, I was a total food addict. I spent my free time eating—mostly inexpensive junk food.

At nineteen, I attempted suicide. There were a number of reasons for that. After assuming I would graduate from college to excel in some fancy profession, I learned that getting straight A's in high school and an immense love of reading didn't automatically translate into a love of college. The lack of structure and lack of interest in general studies classes soon led to me dropping out.

I was working at a video store, eating my parents out of house and home, and failing at life. I had thought life was going to be easy for me (except for the whole secretly Gay thing.) It wasn't. Thanks to God and medical intervention, I obviously survived. I was instantly glad that I did. I was still lost, but I wanted to live.

After about a year of mooching at my beloved grandma's house, a cousin convinced me to go to cosmetology school with her (our moms had been hairstylists all of our lives.) I thought—"Why not?" This was something I knew I could do.

This new direction in my life started me on a path towards so many better things. I was living with my mom again, and she took charge of my food. While in beauty school, I ate only what she made for me. I lost a considerable amount of weight. I made new friends whom automatically assumed that I was Gay. I was busy or tired every day, and the profession forced me to constantly speak to strangers, forcing me to pull myself out of my introversion and learn to comfortably interact with new people.

Once I officially became a hairstylist and officially came out to my new friends, the partying started.

When I turned 21, we started spending weekends at the one local Gay bar (even though it was a dive.) I soon made lots of Gay friends, totally changing the way I saw the world and my place in it.

I was still shy and a bit overweight, so I nervously deflected any opportunities for sex or romance—though to be honest, my chubbiness, somehow greatly magnified by my lack of self-confidence, seemed to prevent most others from being sexually attracted to me. Part of that might have been my lack of experience, causing any interest to go over my head. However, prior to the onset of the "Bear" and "Dad-Bod" movements, I honestly believe that for every excess pound of fat a man carried, his desirability was diminished in kind.

When I became a working hairstylist, I shared a house for the summer with some cohorts from beauty school and a recent Gay pal. We were poor and lived on junk food and alcohol.

It was an amazing time, as I finally developed a social life. We started partying in the large wildly successful Gay nightclubs in the big metropolis about an hour's drive away. Though we were dancing our assess off several times a week, my weight held steady at unpleasingly plump.

After that summer of debauchery (which ended with my virginity still sadly intact,) I moved back in with my parents. Soon I was working in the Kansas City Metro. Still living in a nearby small city, but spending multiple nights per week clubbing with my recently gained Gay friends. I ate my parents' food, and because I didn't pay rent, could indulge regularly in fast food. I quickly regained all the weight I had lost.

As happy as any guy can be whose "not getting any." I settled into a routine.

During these years, I developed really intense infatuations with a few very attractive friends. It was difficult, because the love I had for them (as close friends) was very real, and combined with obsessive physical attraction to them, meant ongoing heartbreak for years. I watched them sleeping around, having one-night-stands, long-term boyfriends, and even dating each other. I remained their much appreciated, but asexual chunky sidekick.

One of them moved across the continent. The other remains a dear friend and was a groomsman in my wedding many years later.

I was, in most ways, happy during these years, despite longing for a personal relationship and a sex life. Eventually, I ballooned to more than a hundred pounds overweight. On my 5 feet, 8 inch frame, that made me obese and almost round. It became almost impossible to see the relatively handsome guy hidden inside the person who now saw a blurry blob in the mirror.

There was a time during those partying years at The Edge, The Cabaret, and The Dixiebell or Sidekicks when I befriended a shorter, very cute little blonde guy. He was clearly crushing on me. We flirted, held hands, and danced at the clubs for weeks.

In retrospect, there was no question that he was sexually and romantically interested in me. Part of me was hesitant to believe it could be true, and another part recognized that the attraction to me was legit—but really without question meant that he had a "fat fetish." He was a *Chubby Chaser*. Later, he would have been thought of just as someone with a thing for Bears—with little or no stigma.

The community was not yet so evolved on such issues. I wasn't personally attracted to overweight men, so I couldn't stand the thought of someone most physically drawn to that aspect of my appearance.

In fact, I faced some backlash from the *in crowd* at The Edge because a very nice and equally obese member of their group had a crush on me for a while and the feeling just wasn't mutual. His friends were offended on his behalf, and didn't enjoy seeing him hurt. I totally understood the feelings of everyone involved, but refused to try to force a relationship that I just wasn't drawn to. Eventually, the Big Guy and I made a sort of friendship, but his popular friends were slower to forgive.

I didn't want someone to love me for being fat when that was the thing I most hated about myself.

Therefore, I began to ignore the Little Guy and give him less attention. Soon, he got the message and faded out of my awareness. He moved on. Later, when I understood myself a little better and could appreciate his interest in me, I began to look for him and hope for another chance, but that ship had sailed. I didn't see him again.

I had a few other opportunities over the years—at least for random sex or one-night stands, but not as many as I expected submerged in a culture of drunk, drugged-out, horny, slutty men for years. I'm not making a generalization about Gay people here, more so, a generalization about nightclub culture. It was pretty hard on an already fragile ego not to be able to just get laid, always immersed in that environment.

Looking back, I see that there were a few (probably way more than I realize) chances that I was just too scared to take. One factor was that despite my desperation, I still had a small, but enduring, seed of dignity and self-respect. I had developed a strong sense of self-worth before I started gaining weight. My ingrained sense of my identity was not that of a fat person, even though it had been my identity for so long.

After almost a decade in the hair industry, I had come out of the closet to my family and met with relative acceptance. The details of that story are for another book.

I followed that career with a decade of work in a quality assurance department of a financial institution. This meant a more steady paycheck, combined with mostly aging out of the party scene.

My weight was increasing, and I had been diabetic for a while. I was inching towards the level of disease that would require taking daily insulin. I had seen what advanced diabetes had done to the health of my grandmother and my dad. I knew it had made my great-grandmother blind. I didn't want my health ruined in that way.

I was also almost thirty, and didn't want to spend my life without a romantic partner. I wanted a shot at love.

My career in the more stable business world meant that I happened to have great medical insurance at the time.

I decided to investigate the nearly unheard of option of bariatric or "weight-loss" surgery. I was desperate enough to gamble with my life, and I made choices that changed everything.

PART TWO

It was around 1999 when I began to research the topic of bariatric (weight-loss) surgery in earnest. I learned what I could online, finally reaching out to one of only about two or three local surgeons with experience and the authority to do weight-loss surgery in my city.

I made an appointment and saw him as soon as possible. The doctor was fairly attractive, hyperactive, and charismatic; in spite of unrestrained arrogance.

I met the requirements of my insurance company of being at least one hundred pounds over-weight and having at least one co-morbidity caused by the obesity. My worsening diabetes, which had been treated until that point with oral medication, met that criterion.

I had to swear that I had tried various diet programs and had taken prescription weight-loss medication. I had taken the moderately successful prescription drug combination popularly known as fen-then (fenfluramine and dexfenfluramine) before the FDA took it off the market in 1997, as it was believed to cause heart valve defects. I was fortunate in that tests showed my heart had not been damaged.

The WL (weight loss) surgeon automatically welcomed me into his program and started planning the surgery with no further testing or even many questions that I recall. It caused me some concern that he didn't want more information, but he could see at a glance how big I was.

All he required to proceed was basically my agreement to follow all of his instructions without question. He expected complete obedience.

The insurance company additionally forced me to have one or two appointments with a psychiatrist. I believe it was his job to see if I understood what I was doing and was likely psychologically capable of embracing the new lifestyle the surgery would require for a successful outcome.

There were booklets and videos I had to watch to prepare for the big day. I had saved up my vacation days and arranged to stay with my parents for a few days to recover.

The surgery took place when I was 30 years old in 2000. It was a desperate act. Many doctors didn't approve of the risk. At the time, I had been told that in the United States, 1 out of 100 bariatric patients dies on the operating table. That meant there was a distinct possibility I might not leave the operating room alive.

My parents had tried hard to convince me that the surgery was too risky. In the end, I convinced them of what I had come to believe myself—that I couldn't lose the weight by myself, and I couldn't go on living as I was. With no other options, my parents agreed to support my decision and to care for me immediately post-op.

I had been put in touch with a few "successful" patients, and I spoke to them briefly on the phone. They assured me that while the path was difficult, the results of the surgery were worth it. I declined to meet with or communicate with the bariatric patient support groups.

I knew they wouldn't put me in contact with anyone whom had a negative experience, and I had already decided that the surgery was my only chance at health and happiness. There was no point, as I saw it, in seeking group consensus—which I sensed would be curated (or highly influenced)—by the cult of personality of my very domineering yet magnetic doctor.

Within a few months, I was admitted to a hospital for the first time in my life; having surgery for the first time in my life. The stress actually caused me to need insulin injections in the hospital—another first which seemed to just confirm the necessity of this life-changing step. I was scared, but mostly hopeful for an exciting new future.

PART THREE

I had no significant other at the time of my surgery, so my parents were there. It's been decades, but as best I can recall, the surgery was a form of *Duodenal Switch*. This type of surgery involved "stomach stapling" to remove much of the stomach and bypass a portion of the intestines. More specifically, the average human stomach holds about 2.5 ounces when empty but expands to hold as much as around 30 ounces when full. In the procedure, the usable stomach is reformed into a small pouch of about one ounce which can expand to hold maybe 2-3 times that amount. The intestine where food exits the stomach is moved and attached to a new outlet, which is intentionally made smaller than normal.

The intention of this is to limit the amount of food the patient can eat at a time to a tiny portion. The smaller outlet means that the food that is consumed will have to exit the stomach very slowly, causing the patient to feel full longer.

Doctors understood at this time (early in the frontier era of bariatric surgery) that after surgery, a frequently occurring problem was that the stomach outlet would gradually dilate or stretch, allowing the patient to eventually begin to eat more again.

In a misguided attempt to work around this predictable problem, which led to weight regain, my surgeon chose to make my new stomach outlet (known as the pylorus) a bit tighter than was customary. I believe he made the diameter of the outlet approximately 2-3 millimeters. Almost no solid food can squeeze through that. Check a ruler. It's about the size of a swollen grain of rice.

The doctor went a step further because even this tiny tube connecting my new little stomach to my intestines would stretch some eventually (which is why so many weight-loss surgery patients at the time would eventually regain most or all of the fat they lost.) With my permission—he was the expert after all—he placed a metal (mesh) ring around the outside of the "new pylorus" to make it impossible for it to ever stretch.

He believed it would almost guarantee that I would never regain any major weight loss. He was correct in his belief that it would prevent the outlet from ever stretching, but neither of us realized what that would really mean.

The surgery itself was pretty brutal. I was sliced open from my sternum down to my belly-button. My entire abdomen was bisected. My ribs were spread, and my abs (abdominal muscles) were cut completely through.

The procedure was performed as he had planned it, with no significant problems. I awoke gagging on the ventilator tube which was still down my nose. The nurses removed it as quickly as possible. It was panic inducing, but normal. Anyone who has ever been on a ventilator would have made every effort, as I did during the pandemic; never to contract Covid.

I was given Morphine and Codeine during and after the surgery. We had no idea that I had an extreme sensitivity to opiates (that we lay persons would call a severe allergy.) I had been told before surgery that it was very important that afterwards I did not vomit under any circumstances. And not to sneeze or cough if I could possibly avoid it.

Almost from the moment I woke up, I was frequently vomiting. It was days before we discovered it was being caused by the opiates, and I was eventually changed to a different class of pain medication.

Obviously, my skin had been stapled together from my chest to my belly-button, and my outer belly (which was slightly deflated) was sort of hanging down and my bruising was so severe that my lower belly region was dark purple because of pooling blood. It was alarming to see. I looked like a monster had torn me open and beaten me.

At that time, I was not allowed to have any food, or even ice or water. I had to be tested to ensure that there were no leaks anywhere in my reconstructed digestive system as that would rapidly lead to infection and possibly then to death.

I was very dehydrated, and whenever I could secretly suck some water from the little sponges (which you are eventually allowed) or swallow a few ice chips; I would immediately start a series of throwing up—though there was nothing to come up but bile. Sometimes it was just dry heaves. Every time could result in something tearing loose inside which, if not immediately found and repaired, would kill me.

For some reason, I felt a strange pressure on my chest. It felt much like when you have a belch stuck in your throat and can't get it out. It's almost like you can't breathe, but it's chest pain at the same time.

Most of the pain was internal, and it's difficult to explain. I had to use a bar above my bed to turn or adjust my body, but that was difficult. I could not ly flat and had been told I would not be able to sleep that way for some time—if ever. I had to sleep with my body elevated to about a 45-degree angle. That's pretty close to sitting upright—only a slight incline.

However, at the time, I couldn't sleep at all. Even after the med change, when I tried to sleep, as soon as I lost consciousness, I would immediately start to vomit. I was being given IVs, but soon felt like I was starving and dying of thirst. I became obsessed with sneaking a few drops of water, despite the danger and knowing the price I would pay.

They almost immediately get you up and force you to start taking walks, so that you won't get blood clots, but I was so weak from no food that I was very shaky on my feet.

It was then that I saw the rooms of some of my surgeon's other patients in this isolated special ward. The nurses and their assistants told me I was lucky to be in the horrific condition I was in. There was a young woman approximately my age whom had essentially the same procedure. I don't know what exactly had gone wrong, but they said she was going to be on a feeding tube for life. I learned he had another weight-loss patient that would be wearing a colostomy bag for life. He had another patient whom while having the same procedure, had died on the table. I would learn other scary details about his patients years later.

Eventually, I was given tiny amounts of water, sugar-free pudding, sugar-free yogurt, an Ensure. None of which stayed down. To add to the frustration, the food staff kept trying to bring me small portions of food. Things I knew I wasn't even supposed to try for several days.

I was taken for X-rays (in a wheelchair) and forced to drink a liquid and try to hold it down for a few minutes to try to get it through most of my digestive system. They also did some kind of MRI or CT scan—all to determine if there were any leaks from my surgical alterations. Eventually, it was determined that by some miracle, there were no leaks.

Meanwhile, I was being given suppositories for the first time, because I wasn't allowed to leave the hospital without having a bowel movement—which had to be caught in a container and inspected and recorded by a nurse. Of course, it had to be the one cute Gay male nurse.

I also had to bathe every day in the shower in my room. I was far too weak to do this by myself. Therefore, my mother had to help me. It was one of the most humiliating things I've ever had to go through. But my mother has never been one to shy away from doing whatever is necessary, and frankly, I had so much pain, fatigue, and weakness that I just complied in whatever way was required and simply let it happen.

I had become so depressed and hopeless, my mind continuously looped between being a totally despondent zombie and panic over the fact that my condition wasn't changing or improving as was usually the norm.

Some of my dearest friends visited, which should have comforted me, but I could see the fear in their eyes when they saw my condition. I'm a very spiritual person, and in my own way, a religious Christian. I began to silently pray constantly. This was not so unusual for me, but it took a dark turn. I stopped praying only to get better, and began to pray that if the way I felt wasn't going to change, that I could just die peacefully. I wanted very much to live, but knew I couldn't bear to go on much longer without improvement.

A couple of very pious friends of my mom's asked when visiting if they could lay hands on me and pray over me. Previously, I would not have been comfortable with such an overt and showy presentation. I always thought it seemed somehow disingenuous. This time, I readily accepted their offer. I cried with the kindness and hope of it. Though I was crying almost constantly in those days.

I was so tired and hungry but could never go to sleep. Once I was allowed to start going for walks by myself, IV in tow, I secretly ventured down to the gift shop. Christmas was fast approaching, and I used money I could not afford to spend to buy very random and over-priced gifts for all of my immediate family because I wanted them to have one last thing to remember me by. I saw no way that I could live until Christmas.

Although I was not remotely fit to go home, after maybe a week, it was determined that I had passed all the required tests and I was sent home.

Initially, I stayed in the home of my dad and his wife. My dad was able to take off work to stay with me for the first several days. The nightmare was just beginning, and my poor parents were terrified and overwhelmed. I was awake around the clock. I had to be sitting up in a recliner at all times. I would pass out from total sleep deprivation, but I was lucky if I slept 1-2 minutes before the vomiting started.

I began to be able to eat popsicles and an ounce or two of water a few times a day. It was a gamble every time I had to take required medications because often they would not stay down.

Soon, I questioned how I was still alive. I was keeping down almost no calories or water for weeks. I thought you could only live like three days without water, and a few more without food. I also believed there was a limit on how many days you could live without sleep; but somehow I lived on. And I was awake. And I was starving.

There was a marathon on TV of the movie *Fried Green Tomatoes*. I watched it twelve times back to back. I thought I was losing my mind. I don't think I was lucid all the time. My step-mom (God bless her.) wanted to return me to the hospital. She also didn't understand how I was still alive.

After a few weeks, I could keep down small amounts of water, Ensure, and saltine crackers (which I dipped in various flavors of salad dressing.) After starving, it seemed like a feast. I had to limit myself to small quantities or I would still throw up. Often, I throw up anyway. But, I was keeping enough down that I could begin to function. I was bathing myself and dressing my incision.

For a while, I continued to stay in my parents' home, though they were gone during the day. I had started to sleep for short periods, as long as I remained almost upright.

We had phoned my surgeon's office frequently with my rather drastic problems, but he and his staff acted as if everything was relatively normal. They were convinced that I was vomiting because I was secretly drinking and eating more than I should have. My parents adamantly assured them I was complying completely with instructions. Our concerns were just dismissed.

After a few weeks or so, I returned to my studio apartment in Kansas City.

By that time, my diet had expanded to include a small bit of peanut butter, but still consisted mostly of crackers with dressing, Ensure, and a little sugar-free pudding or sugar-free yogurt—and popsicles. I had to check labels religiously, because I wasn't allowed to consume anything that included (I think) over 3 grams of sugar per serving.

I was still weak and sleep deprived but was slowly regaining functionality, and I had much less pain. The incision was healing steadily, though the scar alone was disturbing. I had been told to expect having *dumping syndrome,* and I did. That means when I had a bowel movement, it was in the form of diarrhea and that it would cause a drop in electrolytes and fluids; leaving me nauseated, sometimes dizzy, and quite weak immediately after going.

This was frequent. Would occur suddenly and without warning. I was told that it would almost always happen if I consumed even slightly too much sugar, and that I should expect it to be this way for the rest of my life. That was not in the brochure.

I had been blessed to have paid leave from work for all of this time. And my insurance had paid for every penny of the medical expenses. However, soon I had to return to work. I was nervous and embarrassed about the way I now had to live. I had already lost a lot of weight. Maybe 30-40 pounds. I had started at 267. But my butt was almost too sore to walk normally from the constant diarrhea. I was still exhausted. And I was hungry.

Still, it was good to be back at work with my friends, so I packed an extra pair of pants in my backpack (in case of an accident) and went back to my job.

Life became tolerable, and I developed a new normal. I had relatively little pain. I began to eat a few more items; like oatmeal, mashed potatoes, and Jello. Eventually, I even indulged in diet pop. I had occasional follow up office visits with my surgeon. Despite my ongoing complications and problems, he noted my continuing weight loss and declared me a success.

PART FOUR

I had returned to work at my cubicle job, and was glad to have the distraction. Fortunately, my supervisor and co-workers were fairly aware of my situation. There were a couple of large men's bathrooms on our floor, so I could run to the restroom almost immediately as the need frequently occurred. I would often have to be in there for extended periods, and luckily, my employer was very accommodating and understanding. For the most part, it didn't really interfere with my ability to keep up with my work. At least not often.

However, anytime I was leaving my apartment for an extended period of time (to go some place other than work) such as to go shopping, the nightclubs, or some other social occasion; I would postpone eating completely and take an excessive amount of Imodium. It often led to a day or more of constipation, but mostly, it prevented any restroom emergencies while I was out. If I did need to go, I could at least control it.

Over time, I continued to lose weight. I even started to work out at the neighborhood gym every day. Eventually, I lost approximately about a hundred pounds.

I was making new friends, sometimes getting attention or flirtation from men. I was no longer really able to eat at restaurants. At that time, about the only thing I could eat when out was ice cream or pureed soup. At most restaurants, if they have a smooth soup at all, it's tomato. I enjoy that flavor, and sometimes have it, but it is acidic, so sometimes doesn't sit well.

I had been warned, but had not fully understood how much of human interaction revolves around eating—especially at restaurants. I was happy just to go along, but it makes other people (especially in one-on-one situations) uncomfortable for me to sit there watching them as they eat.

In this same period, I realized that the closest I could come to the pleasure of enjoying food was to drink caloric beverages (such as Pepsi or Coke) and eating candy. I've loved candy my whole life, so aside from the sweet taste, it also serves as a comfort item from childhood.

Before long, my desk drawers at work and home were well stocked with a variety of candy and unlimited pop all the time.

In the course of about a year, I had lost one hundred pounds and gained it ALL back. I struggled to believe that I had betrayed myself and all of my suffering; but the proof was on the scale and in the mirror.

I was devastated. Still living with all the negative side effects, and only able to eat a small variety of food items in tiny portions slowly over hours each day. I had to "graze" as my stomach pouch would hold so little food at a time. Even at my lowest weight after surgery, I still had a pretty pronounced belly and chubby face. At no point had my body looked "normal."

After all my weight had returned, I concluded my lifestyle was too horrific to live in that obese body again. I just couldn't force myself to give up the sugar that had recreated it. Already overwhelmed with the constant state of deprivation in which I lived, I couldn't deny myself that small bit of pleasure.

The irony was that the surgery that was supposed to make me healthy made it impossible for me to consume any kind of low calorie nutritious food such as lean meat, vegetables, or fruit. I missed garden salads and apples as much as I missed cheeseburgers. Almost nothing about my surgical experience had gone "as advertised."

So, in my desperation, I took the only help I could find. I called my bariatric surgeon. Had an office visit with him in which I explained everything occurring in my current life.

My state of near hopelessness and his unbridled ego combined to come up with a simple solution.

He would do another surgery on me.

PART FIVE

This surgeon, whom fancied himself a leader in the bariatric surgery community, was not happy with having a failure on his hands. He also thought he could do almost anything and was very comfortable experimenting on his patients—with their consent. He was also a charismatic master manipulator.

In my case, I could usually see through his bullshit from a mile away. However, he and I both knew that when someone is desperate enough, they'll agree to almost anything.

His staff (in this case probably his wife) convinced my insurance company to go all in. This happened almost exactly two years after my first surgery. I was 32 years old when I had the 2nd operation.

What the doctor suggested specifically this time around was that he would remove most of my intestines. They are the organ that processes and absorbs most nutrients and calories from food, so put simply—not much intestine means not much food absorption. It also means saying goodbye to anything remotely resembling a normal bowel movement. What comes out is usually essentially yellow/brown foam. That's what happens when your diet contains little fiber or protein and a lot of fat. None of which is being metabolized in the normal way.

The average adult man has about 21 feet of intestine in total. He would remove all but about 7-9 feet of mine.

He also admitted readily to me (in private) that placing the metal band around the tiny new outlet from my stomach had been a mistake.

The doctor said that while he was removing most of my intestines, he would attempt to remove the metal ring. This would allow the artificial pylorus he had created to slowly stretch and expand some over time. I would be able to eat a more healthy variety of food, and it might put an end to the almost daily vomiting that I suffered.

Let me digress a moment to point out that the vomiting occurred not only when I accidentally (or intentionally) ate too quickly or one more bite than I should. It happened when there was swelling or inflammation in my stomach from previous vomiting, or when I had sinus drainage from a cold or allergies, or sometimes when extra digestive fluids or saliva would build up in my little stomach pouch before it had time to very slowly move into my intestine.

Anyway, he would attempt to remove the metal ring to make my quality of life more tolerable. However, his plan came with a major warning that I had to acknowledge in advance.

Apparently, after weight-loss surgeries like mine, it's not uncommon for adhesions to form around the altered stomach.

Connective tissue causing the surrounding organs to become "stuck" to the stomach or nearby intestines.

Often adhesions form to the liver. The doctor warned that if my liver was stuck to my stomach in the area where the metal ring was located, he would be unable to remove it, as damage to the liver can cause a person to bleed to death very quickly.

As luck would have it, that hypothetical situation proved to be exactly the case (this was confirmed by other doctors later.)

My liver was adhered to my stomach. When the surgeon attempted to raise or move my liver to gain access to the metal ring, my liver immediately started to bleed. He was forced to abandon any attempt to ever remove the metal ring.

He proceeded to remove over half of my intestines, as planned.

I was greatly disappointed, but at least had reason to believe that I would now lose weight again.

My hospital stay was only about three days this time. Though my surgeon was the same, the second operation was performed at a different hospital in the same city. Because we were now aware of my extreme "sensitivity" to certain pain meds, some aspects of the surgery and recovery went more smoothly. Once it was determined that I had no leaks, I was sent home.

This time, I was to recoup in the home of my mom and stepdad. The incision was a bit smaller and make in approximately the same place as the previous one, so the surgical wound itself seemed less traumatic.

Unfortunately, once again, immediately post-op, I could keep nothing down, including liquids and plain water. But this time, that critical issue wasn't being improved by receiving IVs for weeks while recovering in a hospital.

As I experienced the symptoms of dehydration, we called the surgeon's office (hours away from the small town my parents lived in) and were told just to keep trying with ice and water. After a couple of days, I was not only weak and feverish, but becoming delirious. I couldn't think clearly and was struggling to communicate.

My parents got ahold of someone from my surgeon's office and were finally taken seriously. They were told to rush me back to the hospital (2 hours away) where my recent operation had been done.

I was immediately admitted. Because the staff knew I would need multiple IVs, a PIC line was inserted into a major vein in my upper arm. The saline and nutrients soon had me feeling better, but I ended up being kept in the hospital for another week. I feel like this was one of the times I almost died because of these surgeries.

I returned to work sooner this time around. I better understood how I had to eat, which was the same as it was after the first surgery.

I began to lose weight again, but a little more slowly this time. My lifestyle and bathroom issues really didn't change much.

It's important for you to know that by the time I left the hospital after my FIRST surgery, I no longer presented with any of the symptoms or measures of diabetes. That never changed or returned, even after I regained the weight. That is by far the best outcome from the surgeries. Some might argue that makes it worth all the suffering and change in my life, but I can't agree. I'm grateful that the diabetes is "gone," but I've continued to pay a terrible price. There are other ways to manage diabetes.

So life went on. I was back at work. Eating the same. Socializing some, but plagued by my bathroom issues that always had to be at front of mind. I was spending even more time in the bathroom, but for a while I thought I could mange it as I had before. Eventually, I realized the changes to my anatomy in the 2nd surgery were going to prevent me from functioning as I had for the last year. Horror set in as I admitted to myself that everything in my life was going to change.

PART SIX

I didn't want to leave behind the career I had been happy with for a decade. Therefore, my first step was to take short-term disability. I would still be paid, though I was on an extended leave from work.

The situation had left me with no options. Not only was I spending more time at work in the restroom than at my desk, but I was increasingly more certain that it was only a matter of time before I had an *accident* in my pants at work. The anxiety this caused was overwhelming. I could no longer function well enough to do my job, and in those days, I don't think anyone in my company worked from home.

After several weeks with no significant change in my condition, I was able to take "long term disability" from work. It meant reduced pay, but in theory, guaranteed that I would have a job to return to if I were able by the end of the extension.

Instead, as time went on, the long periods in the bathroom left me sore and often experiencing the nausea, dizziness, and general weakness of dumping syndrome. When these episodes happened at night, I could go a day or more at a time without sleeping. I never even knew if I could do a passive activity like reading or writing with any regularity or for a specific amount of time.

I freaked out when I finally had to accept that I wouldn't be returning to the job. It was respectable pay, and I was losing decade old friendships.

Like most people, a lot of my identity, personal self-worth, and dignity, as well as the sense of security tied to the ability to comfortably support myself—were all tied to my career.

I had to apply for Social Security Disability. This meant a great deal of research, collecting physical documentation, and sending lots of faxes, which my apartment's management office was kind enough to let me do.

My first attempt to be approved for Disability was denied despite all the time and work I had put into it while struggling with my medical condition. The research then taught me that my only hope was to engage a Social Security Disability Attorney or Law Firm specializing in cases like mine.

I found a reputable attorney and got a consultation. They were quite reassuring, but they had good news for me and bad.

First of all, because of a backlog in cases, in my area it would take approximately two years to get to go to court. Though they would be working for me behind the scenes during that time, I would not owe them anything until my case was settled. If I won, a specific amount would come out of my first check from the government, which would include back-pay going all the way back to the date I had to leave my job.

In the unusual event that they lost my case, I would owe them some fees, but a plan for that would be determined then. They were motivated to win because it guaranteed them a good paycheck and affected their reputation in this area of specialization.

I dealt with several different lawyers at the firm over the two years, but in the end, it was the older senior partner that represented me in court. I think his personal reputation and vast experience were factors in that decision.

During those two years, I had to see and be examined and tested by three specialists in gastroenterology (none of which could be the shady surgeon that had done my operations.)

These doctors had to provide letters stating my condition, the fact that my condition was unlikely to ever change, and that my condition meant that it would be difficult, if not impossible for me to work outside the home or with any predictable and reliable dependability. The doctors came through with the documentation, and it—along with transcripts of my surgeries from the two hospitals—were passed on to my lawyers.

My future was becoming more uncertain, both in terms of my health and quality of life, but also financially, as I was now living on a fraction of my previous salary.

When the "long term disability" I had through my work ended, and I was officially unemployed, I had regrettably cashed out my modest 401K plan and lived on that money temporarily. When it was gone, I suddenly realized I didn't have next month's rent (which was almost due.) I had a few days to find some place to stay and move out with no notice from the small studio high-rise apartment I had happily called home for 13 years. I was suddenly facing homelessness. Technically, I had been terminated from my job with no warning. It was time to panic.

Because I didn't have time to give proper notice to break my lease correctly (and had just started a new one) I called on all family and friends to help me move, over the course of a weekend, everything it had taken 13 years of living to collect. I had to do this while the management office was closed. They didn't live on site.

The managers already knew of my medical situation and that I had lost my job. Still—I wrote them a long letter explaining why I had to move out immediately, and that I hoped because I had been a good tenet for 13 years, that they would forgive my lease (they would easily re-rent my apartment in weeks for probably twice the rental amount I paid.)

Unfortunately, they chose to enforce the clauses of my lease, meaning that I owed them a few thousand dollars that I could not pay.

They proceeded to report me to the credit companies, making it nearly impossible for me to be approved to rent another apartment and essentially ruining my credit rate until the present day. Twenty years later, my credit is still seriously damaged.

This is another example of the huge destruction to my life resulting from the surgeries and lasting for decades.

Ultimately, I had no options at the time. I was in survival mode.

PART SEVEN

I was blessed to have a lifelong close friend with his own home living in the city. He generously offered to let me stay with him until the outcome of my disability case was determined.

Because I needed to have at least some kind of meager income to pay for my rather specific food needs and some other necessities, our agreement was that along with living in his home for free (his study was temporarily converted to a bedroom for me,) he would pay me 300 dollars a month for acting as his housekeeper—whenever I was able.

At first glance, it seems as if I were very much getting the best end of the deal, but it was complex. I was responsible for running the dishwasher every day and washing some dishes by hand. I did all of his laundry, including ironing his work clothes. I made his bed. I fed his unfriendly cat and changed her litter. On a weekly, and sometimes daily, basis; I swept the floors, dusted, wiped down and watered the indoor plants. I watered the outdoor plants. I cleaned the bathroom probably once a week.

At one point in the height of summer, I was helping prepare the ground and removing old rock patio and lay pavers for a new patio area.

So if you break it down, I was doing all of this work for 10 dollars a day. Yes, I was also given a rent-free room, but as his oldest and closest friend (and considering his well above average income) I would have been highly offended if he actually expected payment from me for having a place to lay my head on a temporary basis.

Our relationship sadly changed for the worse during this time. Previously, we had talked on the phone regularly, went shopping together—essentially shared much of our lives.

While I stayed with him, he gradually stopped conversing with me regularly. He would socialize in the evenings and on weekends with other friends that I didn't really know, and would rarely tell me where he was going and what he was doing. It was odd.

Then, he decided to start trying to control how I spent the 300 bucks he paid me for working in his home. I already used most of it for food, as he intended, but I occasionally used some for music, books, clothes, or going clubbing with other friends. I had to budget it carefully, but never asked him for extra. But, he suddenly went from paying me in cash to getting me a gift card at our local grocery store. It was very controlling, and I did not know what motivated it. It created more of a rift between us.

Fortunately, during this same period, I had a bit of other income. Another friend of mine owned a party bus company, and he "hired me" to answer calls and schedule bookings for parties. It wasn't fun, but it wasn't especially demanding either, beyond the need to be attentive. During the day, I just had to have my computer open to his calendar and listen for the phone calls forwarded to me. It didn't pay much, but it gave me some spending money that was mine to control and allowed me to get out of the house on the weekends.

In the eight to nine months I lived with this dear and old friend, my disability case was progressing. A court date was scheduled, and my attorney prepared me regarding what to expect. My day in court took place in a sort of conference room and was presided over by a judge. The three gastroenterologists, which were our expert witnesses, were all allowed to testify via conference call. This was before the age of Zoom.

The doctors assured the judge that my condition was permeant and that I was not capable of working reliably outside the home, and that I could not even work from home in a way that was dependable or predictable.

The judge ruled I was indeed disabled. I won my case almost exactly two years after we filed. I would receive a hefty back-payment check dating to the time that I was "fired" and begin receiving a monthly check that was much less than I made when working. I learned later that my monthly payment was about the average amount paid to Social Security recipients across the country. Barely enough to live on, but doable.

Because my relationship with my childhood friend (roommate) had so deteriorated by that point, when he asked if I wanted to re-negotiate and continue our living arrangement, I told him with much gratitude for the home he had provided, that I would be moving in with my other best friend whom lived a short distance away in a smaller more modest house. I would pay rent there and would not be the housekeeper; so I would have more rights and freedoms.

The first friend helped me move (along with my family and several other friends.) The semi-wealthy friend was acting normal, and I hoped that returning his privacy to him and normalizing our relationship would heal the discord that had developed between us.

To my continuing sorrow, the opposite happened. As soon as I had completely moved out, he stopped all communication with me. I wrote to him and messaged him, begging for an explanation and apologizing for anything I could have done to offend him. He has never revealed to me the reason why. I have speculated about some possibilities.

He used to leave his valuable watches, his wallet, and wads of cash laying all over the house. If not for me, I think some of it would have been lost, but I usually found everything as I cleaned. I would place it on his bedroom dresser. He may have overheard me on a phone call sometime complaining and bitching about how controlling he had become.

He would definitely have been offended, but I had to vent to others occasionally. He had a rule that I was not to invite any men over for a hookup or to spend the night (even though I had a serious "boyfriend" for a few months during this period.) I was still so shy and inexperienced that aside from dating this one guy for a bit—even though my thinner body was getting more attention—I didn't anticipate that being a problem. However, there was one Saturday night that I let a cute guy drive me home after the club. I invited him to spend the night because he was really too intoxicated to be driving, and it was only hours until morning.

We went to bed and played around a little before falling asleep. Early the next morning, my roomie made a point of letting me know he knew the guy was in my room and that he was not happy about it. It was humiliating, and I basically had to kick the man out. I got the silent treatment for a while and then a lecture. I was incredibly insulted.

My mom, whom had known the roommate since he was born, suspected that he might have had a crush on me and been jealous and later offended when I moved out.

While I think that's a possibility, I wasn't really his type, and we had grown so distant. I don't think that was it.

So, I don't know if he thought I stole from him; he overheard me talking about him in anger, if he thought I should pay him back-rent (even though I had really been a poorly paid live-in servant,) or if there was possibly romantic feelings, or something else entirely.

I have attempted contact at several key moments over the years, but he has never acknowledged me or explained. I miss him terribly and always will. I would be thrilled to put it all behind us if he would ever reach out, but I have little hope anymore.

I have shared the great generosity and tragic outcome of this time period, because I feel that losing my closest and oldest friend was one of the greatest costs of having these life-ruining surgeries.

I quit working for my friend with the bus business, whom really didn't need me, and had mostly helped me out of pity, and settled into my tiny bedroom in my other BFFs little home.

I used my lump some check to pay off a few debts, buy some much needed furniture, get a new computer, and my first cell phone—and a cat. I needed a wardrobe for my new smaller body, so before long, most of the lump payment was gone.

Did I mention that a person going on disability does not qualify for Medicare until two years after they start being paid by Social Security? So, I was without health insurance for the first time in my life. That was scary, but fortunately, I had no big medical expenses during that period. I was using over-the-counter medications to try to moderate the symptoms of my botched surgeries. Or more accurately, surgeries performed correctly (though executed in an extreme way) but with devastating results.

The guy I had been dating through the Autumn months dumped me immediately after helping me move, but within a few weeks I had started dating my first REAL boyfriend.

In the period of a few months, almost everything in my life had changed—AGAIN, but I was happy. I still struggled with all the surgery related challenges, but my life was interesting. And fun.

PART EIGHT

So began my first serious relationship and three years of living with the best friend I had since becoming an adult.

I had been walking daily to encourage continued weight loss, because as severe as my surgeries had been, exercise was still required for the loss to continue. I was no longer interested in going to a gym, but long walks allowed me to listen to music or often audio-books.

A great perk of my new living arrangement was that we live next to a very cool walking trail that wound through pleasant neighborhoods, which provided for great people watching.

Soon I was spending about one week at home, then spending one-two weeks at my boyfriend's home. I took my cat with me.

My life was greatly improved for a while. My complicated bathroom needs were embarrassing—both with my new roomie and his constant string of boyfriends and my own boyfriend (whom I didn't want to be grossed out.)

My continued complicated food needs meant keeping my own food on hand at home, and having food at my boyfriend's house. That got expensive fast. That meant my boyfriend usually paid for my food at his place. Something that he grew to resent over time despite his generous nature.

It is all just a lot for people to deal with. At that time, no one I knew had experience with people whom had such surgeries, and they understood even less about everything that had gone wrong for me and what complications it meant in my daily life.

Which foods worked for me could seem very random, and the fact that so often none of these worked for me was hard to understand. I think it would be hard for people to believe that it was all totally real. That I wasn't exaggerating.

Soon, I was spending most of my time at my boyfriend's house. It was as if I were spending 400 dollars per month for a small storage unit at my friend's place. I tried to convince my sweet boyfriend that it was time to take the next step. That I should move in with him, which would allow me to use any excess funds to get my own groceries and help with expenses at my boyfriend's place.

Unfortunately, he declined. My feelings were hurt, and a wedge was driven between us. Darren's explanation was that he didn't feel completely secure in our relationship. He was afraid that if it didn't work out between us, I would be left having a difficult time to find a place I could afford on my own. I would be stuck.

His logic was sound, but I had hoped he would have enough faith in us to believe that we could make it.

I couldn't see remaining in the status quo if we weren't headed towards something more serious. That's when I came to the sad conclusion that we had to break up. Whether real divination or a lucky guess—the Tarot reader we had encountered at Pride Fest early in our relationship had been right about our time together being short term. After two years, I was single again. For the last year I lived with my old friend, I was home most of the time, which cramped his style a bit and got on his nerves.

Luckily, our friendship was saved from further damage, when a good friend of my mom's (whom happened to manage my hometown's low-income apartment complex—which was mostly for senior citizens) let me know she had a one-bedroom unit opening in a few months. I had to formally apply, but if I wanted it, it was mine.

I really wasn't mentally prepared to move back to my tiny hometown. At this point, I had lived almost my entire adult life (around 25 years) in Kansas City. There was a thriving LGBTQ Community. To my knowledge, there was one openly Gay person in my hometown—and he was a teenager.

I didn't want to leave city life behind. I still remembered all too well what it could be like for Gay people in a rural environment. But I wasn't afraid anymore. I wasn't feeling especially social, and the idea of spending more time with my aging parents and watching my nephews finish growing up was appealing. Besides, I looked forward to having my own place again.

Moving was a pain in the ass, as it always is but I liked my new reasonably spacious apartment. I would miss my special walking trail, but I could walk around the town (literally) when the mood struck. My familiar (cat) was kind of bored without other people and animals around, so I soon acquired a "care kitten" to be his companion.

We settled in and it was a nice, quiet private life. I only occasionally missed getting out and about. It was awkward being the town's token inked and out Gay, but my family and I knew most of the villagers, so it wasn't a totally alien environment.

I got called "that Gay guy" by a three-year-old while returning from my mailbox. And there were several months when someone pounded on my door in the middle of the night—I was always disappointed by the time I could open it (butcher knife in hand for protection.) That happened a few times a week for a few months. It was pretty scary, but I figured it was kids pulling pranks. It became much more frightening when it escalated to someone using BBs to shoot a hole through my living room window (breaking it.) Nearly hitting my cat and only missing me by a few feet.

It was kind of humiliating having to report these events to the local cop. He took a report and examined my windows and seemed to take the situation seriously. However, he warned me that unfortunately, there wasn't much he could do unless someone was caught in the act.

You may ask yourself why I'm telling you about homophobic harassment.

It's because so much of the path my life took and the choices I was forced to make, have directly resulted from my extreme surgeries and their repercussions.

The complications and resulting disability put me in positions and situations that would never have occurred if I had not had those cursed surgeries.

Still, life in my family's town was pleasant in many ways. I actually lost a lot of additional weight over my time there. I actually got down to my personal goal weight of 145 pounds for a while.

My belly was saggy (despite a fatty lipoma in my abdomen that prevented my stomach from ever being flat.) My butt (while flat) was saggy, as were my skinny thighs. My arms were a bit floppy, and my deflated chest (while I didn't have man boobs) sat strangely low on my body. My face somehow looked almost skeletal while still looking too big. I have this naturally wide jaw bone, combined with sort of muscular cheeks.

Over all though, I looked pretty attractive in clothes (and even naked, if I could hide my saggy belly.) Let me note here that many people, after extreme weight loss, seek cosmetic surgery. At least a tummy tuck, if not a full body lift. My understanding has always been that because these surgeries are cosmetic, insurance rarely pays for them unless the excess skin is causing some other serious medical condition (such as yeast infections recurring within the skin folds.) I had no such conditions, and am somewhat terrified of surgery at this point. Also, if this excess skin is removed, if the weight is later regained, you may face a whole new set of serious problems.

A lot of people seemed to want me, but no one remotely in my area. The few that were within a reasonable proximity were all married closet cases. I wasn't into that, so my dating life was nearly non-existent for about 5 years.

The sad truth is, I had inadvertently reached my weight goal almost accidentally. My weight had held steady for years at around 165 pounds—approximately one hundred pounds below my highest weight.

At first I didn't realize what had changed in my lifestyle that had made the additional weight loss possible.

In the privacy of living alone, I had developed a habit that became more extreme over time. I allowed myself to binge on foods that I knew my stomach couldn't possibly keep down. All the delicious things that I had denied myself for so long.

It's not a pretty story, but this is what happened. I would prepare a feast of various favorite foods, then splurge as quickly as I could eat. I knew I would only have 5-10 minutes before the pain and discomfort would become so great that the undigested food would all have to come back up. In my head, I called those items bucket food, because I would have to throw it all up into a bucket, which I then emptied into the toilet. It was all super gross. It didn't really taste bad, because it came up mostly in the same condition it had gone down, but it didn't smell good, and it looked disgusting.

Cheeseburgers, pizza, baked chicken, mac-n-cheese, big sandwiches. I did it all. Everything that had been impossible for decades. It was my darkest secret. I had essentially become bulimic, though I never thought of it that way.

Eventually, I did it so much that the food shopping and preparation consumed most of my time. Add to that the time I spent eating and vomiting, and afterwards I was too depleted and tired to prepare or even eat the foods I could actually keep down for nourishment.

Also, usually after hours of binging and puking, nothing else I ate (or even drank would stay down.) I had to sleep several hours first. It was like sleep would reset my stomach and usually it would function in my normal way by the next day. Often I would just rehydrate and have a yogurt or something and then start the binging and purging cycle all over again. I was honest enough with myself to be embarrassed, but I still didn't consciously think of it as bulimia.

PART NINE

Probably four years into my return to single small-town life, I experienced an alarming medical crisis.

I often kept odd sleeping patterns, because I love to stay up all night watching TV, reading, looking at social media, talking to guys on Grindr, etc. I would then sleep most of the next day. I had been a night owl all of my life, and always stayed up as late as I could. Too late, when I was working, but I managed it.

After too many days of sleep deprivation, it wasn't unusual for me to spend a few days mostly sleeping to "catch up." Other than annoying my cats, it really wasn't a problem (and I still didn't miss their feedings.)

However, I found myself in the unusual circumstances of having slept about four days without having the energy to get up and bathe or eat. I barely had the strength to go to the bathroom and get some juice or water from the fridge. By the time I cared for the cats, I was back in bed, passing out.

Eventually, I realized this was abnormal, and I was scared. I went to the doctor. They took a blood sample and gave me a cup for a fecal sample. When the tests came back, my doctor was panicked (this was my family physician—not the shady surgeon.) The stool sample showed only the normal trace amounts of blood, but they feared I might be bleeding internally. My red blood cell counts (for which I think around 14 is the norm) were down to like a two. Red cells carry oxygen to all parts of your body, including your brain. My doctor and his staff were left wondering how I was conscious and how I was walking and moving around. My life was in imminent danger. I needed iron. A sufficient level of iron is necessary for our bodies to make red blood cells.

Normally, our food is an adequate source of iron. Our bodies even store enough extra to last quite sometime. However, sometimes people need to take supplements.

I had been instructed to take multi-vitamins immediately after surgery—which would include iron. I could never do so. Iron taken orally caused me severe constipation. I had taken almost no vitamins because the outlet from my stomach had been made so small that they would get stuck. For years post surgery, I had to use a pill cutter/crusher to take any medication that wasn't liquid. My blood work had shown my vitamin levels somehow within the normal range for many years, so I had stopped worrying about it.

But suddenly, my iron stores were gone. I had to go to the nearby cancer/hematology center to be given iron infusions.

It was so bizarre. The nurses would have to slowly inject like a pint of this black sludge (iron) directly into my veins. At this time, because of my low income (I actually qualified for 16 dollars a month in food stamps) the hospital actually wrote off any medical expenses that I had which were not covered by Medicare. These treatments would have been expensive, but they cost me nothing.

I had to be infused every week for 5 weeks, then my levels were tested. My iron and red cell count was slowly going up, but it took three of those 5 week rounds to get me to an acceptable level.

After that, I had to do another round maybe every three months. Finally, my levels stabilized.

It has now been five years since my last infusion. I still see the hematologist about three times per year. They check my iron and red cell levels, as well as a few other relevant blood factors. The red cell levels have been remaining fairly steady close to normal, but the iron level is very slowly dropping. Eventually, I will require another infusion. This will probably be required at least every few years or so for the remainder of my life. Chronic and extreme anemia is a scary and dangerous thing.

PART TEN

Eventually, I met a man. The man I would later marry.

We met online, then in neutral territory—a nearby shopping mall.

Both of us were pretty thin at the time. Him, because he was a college student over 20 years my junior and living on ice cream, cocktails, and an empty fridge.

Me, for all the reasons I've just explained. It took time, and curiosity for him to understand my bizarre lifestyle, my diet, and the reasons for it.

Months later, we were engaged, and after more than a year, we were married. The last time I needed an iron infusion was a week before our wedding. My lab numbers have held up well since, but are in slow decline. I will need another infusion of black sludge, eventually. The next time around, and every time after, I'll be paying for whatever portion my insurance doesn't cover.

Eating habits changed for each of us after marrying. Though my husband had success with Weight Watchers during our engagement, we both began to put on the traditional weight after we wed. Married life means staying home in front of the TV most evenings, which for most people means weight gain. My husband has dieted off and on over the last 5 years with varying degrees of success.

I haven't really tried to diet. I feel like I am already denied the pleasure of most food. Variety and healthy food choices are almost non-existent, so it is difficult to deny myself even further.

The most critical change for me is that because I now live in close quarters with another person and our combined limited incomes have to pay all the bills; it is too irresponsible, unfair, and grotesque for me to continue the habit of binging and purging.

I now only try to eat foods I believe I will probably keep down. That isn't always successful. No matter how careful I am, I sometimes still throw up daily. Other times, I can go weeks with everything staying down.

He appreciates that I try, and pities me when it doesn't work. At first, it really grossed him out, but he now understands that it is largely beyond my control. Sometimes it only takes one bite of a food that usually works very well for me to start the vomiting. Sometimes it starts BEFORE I've had a single bite.

Socializing is difficult, because it's hard to dine out with friends or family when almost the only thing I can eat from a restaurant is smoothly pureed soup (only consistently available at one chain restaurant,) mashed potatoes (though it's hard to find them without skins unless the place serves the instant form,) or desserts including ice cream. These criteria eliminate almost all fast food, which is really all our budget allows with any frequency.

Yet, for all of these limitations, the few staples that I CAN eat are high in fat and sugar.

I am still addicted to candy and pop. Occasionally, I go through periods of sticking to diet pop, but usually return to my full sugar favorites. I also love myself some sports drinks and Snapple—I don't choose diet with those either.

As a result, during my marriage, I have gained back about 55 pounds. Still well below my all-time high, but moving in that direction. Strangely, my belly seems bigger than ever.

My hope is that we can both get a handle on it and lose a healthy amount. I no longer feel the need to be thin. I just want to be healthy and look decent in normal clothes. Basically, be generally in control and more human shaped so that I am more physically comfortable and feel a bit more attractive. It's attainable with a little more self-discipline.

We briefly both tried intermittent fasting. On some days we do it naturally, so it seemed doable, and the science behind it makes complete sense. However, we both found it surprisingly hard to stick to when it was intentional.

My husband will probably be most successful with what has worked for him in the past—doing Weight Watchers and using an app to track daily points which are assigned to specific foods and portion sizes.

Because my food choices are so limited, and I have to kind of slowly graze almost all day for the food to stay down, that system won't work for me.

I think my best hope will be cutting out as much sugar as possible, portion control, and the elimination of snacking. Wish me luck. I know it will be a lifelong struggle.

Some last information I want to share with you includes that I now must take a large amount of Nexium every day in an attempt to control acid reflux. I sleep in an adjustable bed so that my upper body can be elevated. I take low dose pain meds daily to deal with mysterious abdominal pain. It's kind of stabby, so I feel like it may be related to the metal staples in my stomach, but who knows? I sometimes have to take the same anti-nausea meds that chemo patients take to try to keep my food down. My butt sometimes becomes so sore from extended time on the toilet that I have to take a small handful of Ibuprofen to reduce the inflammation (despite the potential damage to my liver or stomach lining.) I finally developed my first hemorrhoid a few months ago. That was a nightmare, but I'm sure there are more of those in my future. I should mention I also lived with an "anal fissure" for a while. Think of it as a painful tear in the rectum that is slow to heal and feels like fire every time you go to the bathroom.

As you can imagine, there are many parts of this lifestyle that are anxiety inducing. This eventually led to occasional panic attacks. These were a horrific revelation to me, because I usually am not even experiencing stress when they happen. To prevent these from occurring regularly and to control them when they do, I now take daily meds for anxiety too.

You need to know a bit more about my diet.

First off, I was told before my surgeries that within days, I would be eating things like eggs, bacon, peanut butter—and then, within a few weeks, small portions of almost anything.

None of that happened.

I explained earlier what my post surgery diet was like. It was several years before I could sometimes keep down a poached or scrambled egg—it's still a gamble. Eventually, I could eat a slice or two of crispy bacon, though it also doesn't always work. I still don't try them in public.

My typical diet 20 years after my surgery includes the following on a regular basis: cheese, yogurt (with no firm fruit chunks,) mashed potatoes, tuna with mayo, crab with mayo, crackers, potato chips, dip, humus, tortilla chips, salsa (that isn't too chunky,) Jello, ice cream, canned cream soup, canned green beans, peanut butter/jelly (without bread,) over-cooked rice, over-cooked Ramen noodles cut into tiny pieces, popsicles, Ensure, cookies, oatmeal (thinned out,) applesauce, and pudding. That's pretty much it.

Ironically, even though I had the surgeries to lose weight and be more healthy; I can eat almost no fiber or fresh produce (or really almost any solid fruit or vegetable,) no salad, no red meat (only fish or chicken in shredded form,) no bread or pasta. I don't tolerate milk well, or tea, or black coffee. I never dreamed I would spend most of my life fantasizing about a garden salad.

Desserts usually work for me because they are made up mostly of fat and sugar. They melt.

You may be thinking that some things that usually agree with me are pretty tasty—even delicious—and they are. They are also pretty fattening and offer little nutrients. Imagine, even the most yummy things on my "yes" list making up every meal, every day for 20 years, and going forward for the rest of my life.

I must also note (again) that sinus drainage, whether caused by infection or allergies, is not my friend. It often has the effect of pooling in my stomach pouch more quickly than it can pass through. This can cause random nausea and vomiting, sometimes for days.

You may wonder if there are some surgical options to correct my anatomy and make it possible to live a more ordinary life.

According to my gastroenterologist, the answer is no.

The only surgical option would be to attempt to make a NEW outlet from my stomach, ignoring the present highly restrictive outlet. My intestines would then be moved and attached to this new hole in my stomach. The specialists strongly advised against it because of the danger. Just getting to the outside of my stomach would be dangerous because of my liver being adhered to it, and any time you are making a hole in the stomach and disconnecting / moving the connection of the intestines, it's possible for leakage to occur before healing is complete. That can be deadly. On top of that risk, the best-case scenario was that I might be able to eat slightly more food, or slightly faster, or gain some variety in the foods I can eat.

It is also possible that such a surgery could go smoothly, and there would still be no improvement in my ability to eat. It's just not worth the risk. Not even maybe. There has been more than enough experimentation done on my internal anatomy. I also have too much to live for to place my life in that kind of jeopardy again.

So I will just be grateful for my situation. I'm alive. I don't require a feeding tube. I can eat a small but tasty variety of foods. I still remind myself of the weeks after my surgeries, when I prayed desperately, that I could someday drink water again without carefully sipping and limiting it. I have that now, so I'm blessed.

Soon after my second surgery, my young surgeon died suddenly of an undetected heart defect. Or at least that was the public story. He left behind a wife and kids. I learned at that time that there were six bariatric surgery related lawsuits against him at the time of his death. I'm guessing that the girl with the permanent feeding tube and the patient that had died on the operating table were two of those.

Several people thought I should sue his estate. There was no doubt that he had done permanent and extreme damage to my quality of life and ability to support myself—partially through experimental surgical techniques. However, the other surgical specialists that had examined me later had stated that my deceased doctor had not actually made any mistakes in my surgery. He had simply altered my anatomy to a slightly more severe degree than was customary. Part of my complications were just the unpredictable way my body had reacted to the surgery. Based on their expert analysis, I might have lost my case anyway. In retrospect, I should have tried. I deserved that compensation. At least aspects of my life today would be easier, if I had won.

Today, bariatric surgeries have become much more advanced. I recognize that most weight-loss procedures done now are considered less invasive and usually (in theory—reversible.)

There is the gastric sleeve, Lap-Band, biliopancreatic diversion, gastric bypass, and others. Some of these can even be done laparoscopically. However, some are still very similar to what was done to me. Despite some procedures being advertised as reversible, I have met no one whom has had their procedure reversed.

Some of these procedures result in less weight loss because the alterations are less extreme and the patient can eat somewhat normally.

Of course, slower or less total weight loss can result in less satisfaction for the patient. Anecdotally, I have heard of mixed results. Many patients do experience significant weight loss with these updated procedures, with side effects they consider being worth the result. How long the weight loss is maintained varies, with the success often depending on how well the patient has learned the self-discipline necessary to make better food choices and maintain portion control.

However, I know that some patients, particularly those having procedures similar to mine, end up living with complications similar to some of mine—often including eventually regaining the weight.

I strongly advise most people considering weight-loss surgery against it. I'm not a medical professional, but I am an experienced guinea pig—I mean patient. I am a cautionary tale.

With family members and friends whom have considered bariatric surgery, I have strongly campaigned against it. My argument is simple: Why risk your life and severe complications by mutilating your body, when to achieve the desired results; post-surgery, you will still be forced to greatly alter and restrict your diet and adhere to an exercise program to achieve major weight loss and maintain it over time?

Although the surgery will force the alteration in your diet, you will still feel the constant hunger, still miss all the social aspects of eating with people (especially in public,) you will still sacrifice most of your favorite foods, in order to reach your goals.

If you can deal with that hunger, the extreme lifestyle changes, and the restricted food choices; you might as well make those changes without having surgery. You will get the same results without the trauma and damage to your body.

There are some especially extreme cases, when I would actually suggest weight loss surgery despite the danger.

If a person's obesity has led to such advanced diabetes, they are experiencing neuropathy, possible blindness or other severe damage; they have nothing to lose by trying the surgery.

If a person is so obese, that they can not drive or fit in a car, if they can not be supported by regular furniture, if they can not walk un-assisted because of their size—they should definitely have the surgery if their doctor approves.

If a person's life or health is worse than my compromised and very damaged quality of life, it seems like bariatric surgery would almost certainly IMPROVE their life. It's worth taking the chance… if their doctors agree.

IN CLOSING

I wrote this book for the many people that are in the situation I was in. I was fat. I was diabetic. I didn't like the way I looked. (The Gay community can be especially critical and judgmental about appearances.) I felt I could never discipline myself enough to make the change necessary to save myself.

What I thought would be the easy way to be thinner and more fit proved to create as much suffering as I was trying to avoid and much more.

So, as I live with my disabilities, struggles, and medical issues, I will continue to try to lose weight and be healthier. And I will have to do it the old-fashioned way. Deny myself my favorites. Stop eating while I'm still hungry. Try to move more. All the same things I needed to do before I had surgery.

So, research, talk to as many post-op patients as possible (not just those your doctor refers you to) and read everything you can. Unless your obesity is already crippling you, have the least invasive, least restrictive procedure possible, and have reasonable expectations. Know that you will still have to do most of the work. You will still be hungry, and you will always crave the delicious foods that made you fat.

Lastly, please consider other options. Even though you may feel you have already tried them all. If my life, as I have described it, would be better than the life you're living now, a well-planned surgery may indeed be the best answer for you.

If my story causes you to hesitate, please continue to try the traditional ways of losing weight. Try to eat un-processed food, control portion size. Accept help wherever you can get it. I wish you luck. Please send some my way in return.

Being fat is hard. Losing weight is harder. Sometimes living with bad choices is the hardest of all.

AUTHOR BIO

Silas Scott is an author of topic specific memoirs about many of the profound aspects of his life that are unique and unusual while somehow being relevant and really important to lots of other people. He is a married, middle-aged Gay man from the Midwest sharing the events, meaning, and wonder of his life filled with spirituality and a lifetime of struggling to be comfortable in his body. Too shy to speak his truths, he expressed his reality and dreams through drawing and writing. As a man of nearly 50, he found he had to use his empathy and words to fight for social justice, equality, and self-actualization for himself and all LGBTQ people in front of politicians, church elders, newspaper reporters, and TV cameras. Mr. Scott's daily joy comes from reading, laughing with his husband, and caring for their beloved pets. Mr. Scott was a pretty boy that grew into a fat young man, forever battling to be healthy and comfortable in his own skin. Check out his soon-to-be-released other non-fiction books about the most personal subjects that people hesitate to talk about but that most powerfully affect our lives.

IF YOU WOULD BE SO KIND

I hope you found this book informative and enjoyable. It is meant to share parts of my life in order to allow you to better understand people like me. To better understand yourself, your family member, your co-worker, classmate, neighbor, or friend—whom may be struggling with being over-weight; and the extreme risks involved in Weight Loss Surgery.

Please look for my other forthcoming memoirs about topical personal issues that may help you to better understand yourself or others.

Please share a fair review of tis book wherever you buy or talk about books.

Check out my website to learn more about the issues that matter in my life and that may be important to you.

Website: silasscottauthor.com

www.ingramcontent.com/pod-product-compliance
Lightning Source LLC
Chambersburg PA
CBHW071145240526
45465CB00024BA/1784